T0126933

66 DAY JOURNAL

66 DAY JOURNAL

A GUIDED JOURNAL FOR CREATING NEW HABITS

MATTHEW MOCKRIDGE

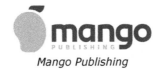

Mango Publishing

Copyright © 2019 Matthew Mockridge
Published by Mango Publishing Group, a division of Mango Media Inc.

Cover Design: Jayoung Hong
Illustrations: Jayoung Hong
Layout: Jayoung Hong
Editing: Doris Eichhorn-Zeller

Mango is an active supporter of authors' rights to free speech and artistic expression in their books. The purpose of copyright is to encourage authors to produce exceptional works that enrich our culture and our open society.

Uploading or distributing photos, scans or any content from this book without prior permission is theft of the author's intellectual property. Please honor the author's work as you would your own. Thank you in advance for respecting our author's rights.

For permission requests, please contact the publisher at:
Mango Publishing Group
2850 S Douglas Road, 2nd Floor
Coral Gables, FL 33134 USA
info@mango.bz

For special orders, quantity sales, course adoptions and corporate sales, please email the publisher at sales@mango.bz. For trade and wholesale sales, please contact Ingram Publisher Services at customer.service@ingramcontent.com or +1.800.509.4887.

66 Day Journal: A Guided Journal for Creating New Habits

ISBN: (p) 978-1-64250-158-2, (e) 978-1-64250-159-9
BISAC category code GAM021000, GAMES & ACTIVITIES / Guided Journals

Printed in the United States of America

"

This journal belongs to _____

This is my journal number ____

For the time period of _____ to _____

If you are working toward a goal with a partner,
here is some space for a few encouraging words from him/her:

"

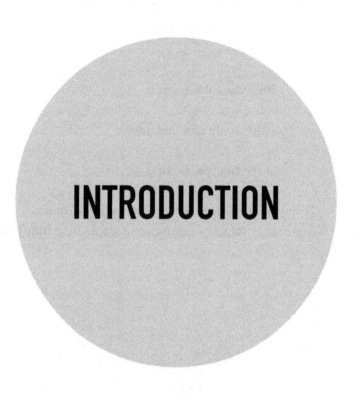

INTRODUCTION

• Why This Journal Works •

Deconstructing

Sometimes achieving a goal can be quite difficult. However, a goal is just many parts put together. With the help of this journal, we will disassemble these parts into 66 mini-projects, which will lead you to completing your goal!

Incentive

Motivation is an overused term. Everyone has days when they are not motivated and just want to watch Netflix all day long. It's normal, I promise you! The *66 Day Journal* uses the latest insights taken from behavioral and positive psychology and neuroscience—as well as the patterns and techniques commonly used by most super performers in fields ranging from professional sports, entertainment, and business—to help us be more motivated!

Automation

The continuous repetition of an action becomes automatic after 66 days. Achieving a goal is only the beginning! The *66 Day Journal* is designed to help you create and firmly integrate new routines into your everyday life. Routines that are needed to reach your greatest goals, all without having to think about the process, thus protecting your decision-making power.

How This Journal Works

The *66 Day Journal* is your training partner. For the next 66 days, you will be systematically guided every day to achieve your goal.

• How to Set a Goal •

The SMART theory, developed by Peter Drucker, uses five pillars contained in every well-set goal:

S–Specific

M–Measurable

A–Attainable

R–Relevant

T–Time Bound

Specific

What exactly do you want to achieve? Clear actionable steps can only be determined if you can name the specific details of your target.

Measurable

Only goals that are measurable can be definitively achieved. The more specifically you can define key figures and components of your target, the better your chances of success will be.

Attainable

Keep it real to avoid frustration! Even just landing some jabs will carry you through the rounds of your toughest battles. Big goals are important, but make sure your goals are not unrealistic.

Relevant

Is your goal useful and valuable to humanity? Is it important to you? *Real* relevance gives you honest conviction!

Time Bound

If there is no deadline, there is no end point. Using this journal, your window of time is clearly defined—66 days.

• Finding Your Passion •

1. Look Behind Your Biggest Fear.

Do what frightens you the most, and you will find your passion. Simply feel the fear, and do it anyway! The feeling that you get when you are coming out the other side of your fear is real passion generated through real pride.

2. Passion Comes AFTER Practice, Not Before.

Many people think that they have to find their passion first in order to find the strength to exercise regularly. In fact, it's the other way around! Focusing on the practice regimen will lead to the emergence of true passion, while generating honest fulfillment through steady growth. Work to become good at something, and you'll be passionate about it.

3. Practice Properly.

Practice what is most difficult! World-class musicians always repeat the most difficult parts of the song. Mediocre musicians like to play the whole song, usually songs they already play well. True growth happens when you practice the parts you want to practice the least—the hardest parts.

4. What if Money Wasn't Important

If you were financially independent tomorrow, what would you do? Taking the monetary variable out of the equation always reveals true passion.

5. What Did You Always Want to Do as a Child?

All the dreams you had before someone told you that you were not allowed to live them are always close to your passion. If you can't remember what you always wanted to do as a child, just talk to people you have known for a long time. They might see things in you that you might not be able to see in yourself anymore. Your best friend from the third grade, your grandparents, your siblings, etc.

6. Find Your Valuable Places.

Look for places that put you in a creative state. These places and their attributes are often very precise indicators of the places that are closest to your passion.

• The Questions Used in This Journal •

The quality of your questions determines the quality of your life!
The questions used in this journal combine mindfulness, positive
psychology, and proven strategies for increased productivity.

1. What Am I Proud Of?

Feeling proud is a powerful tool. Don't wait until you pass the finish
line to be truly proud of yourself. Finding your pride is necessary to
increase your productivity. During this journey of finding what makes
you proud, make sure you reflect deeply every step of the way—this will
give you joy and energy.

2. Three Things I Am Thankful For (Three New Things Every Day):

Find new things to be thankful for every day and gradually refocus the
lens through which you see the world. By regularly looking for all that
is good in your life, you will begin to see endless potential where others
only see annoying problems.

3. What I Am Happy About in My Life Right Now?

Through the effects of "hedonic adaptation" the luxury of today
becomes the standard of tomorrow. People get used to nice things very
quickly and loose the ability to be truly happy. The daily reflection on
your happiness has the power to reawaken your joy instantaneously.

4. Notes/Thoughts:

All cognitive processes that occur in your mind without you even
noticing cost you an ever increasing cognitive tax and dangerously blur
the clarity of your vision. "Downloading your thoughts" moves
these processes from mind to paper, creating space for your most
meaningful work and your most important goals.

5. What Did I Learn Today?

Through daily repetition, you have the ability to heavily manipulate your learning curve. As soon as you regularly reflect on your most valuable insights you will lock them in forever.

6. What Could I Have Done Better?

What isn't measured isn't improved! It is important to try to write and frame the answer to this question as a positive, new reality. Don't write, "I could have lost less time watching TV!" Instead, write, "I don't watch TV!" In this way, a potential frustration is turned into a solid implementation of a totally new and valuable behavior.

7. The "Big Points" I Will Achieve Today, in Order to Progress in My Goal:

What isn't scheduled doesn't get done. Your daily "Big Points" make you responsible for yourself. Our daily progression is now easily trackable.

8. For the Next Sixty-Five Days I Will...and in Sixty-Five Days I Have

Visualization is the invaluable ability to see things before they have happened. The mind *knows* the situation because it has *seen it* in thought. Professional athletes, successful entrepreneurs, and famous artists all use this insight in order to achieve their most important goals and allow their visions to come to life.

9. Three Amazing Things that Happened Today?

Who were you able to help, what gave you joy, what felt beautiful? If you look after your most precious moments, your happiness will take care of itself. Reflecting on three amazing, touching moments of your day allows you to relive the experience and feel what you felt. Sharing these special moments with others multiplies their power.

• Goal Example •

Goal: I want to lose five kg in 66 days!

Specific:

I want to lose at least five kg in the next 66 days through the low carb diet method and three training units per week. I will train at my local gym and jog three times a week on my favorite trail in the woods. My best friend is my training partner!

Measurable:

I have calculated my calorie requirement, and I know that I cannot consume more than two thousand calories per day. I can document my training progress and record my body weight development daily.

Attainable:

I have enough time to go to the gym three times a week and jog three times a week. I will use the time that I would otherwise have used for watching television. I can stay within my calorie requirement as long as I decide to purchase healthy food while grocery shopping. The decision is made while shopping, not while looking in the fridge.

Relevant:

I want to improve my health and self-esteem in order to be a good example for my family and my community.

Time Bound:

My goal is to go to the gym three times a week and jog three times a week all for 66 days.

Do it today, not tomorrow! The next 66 days will pass with or without your full commitment toward the realization of your goal! Telling a lot of people about your goal creates responsibility and accountability. It also inspires others to pursue their goals!

Get another person on board whose growth you believe in and experience the next 66 days as accountability partners. Help each other with the implementation of your routines and be responsible for each other.

Whether you start alone or as part of a team, if you use the unbelievably powerful mechanics of this journal correctly, you *will* reach your goal!

• My Goal •

Now you try. Outline your own goal based off the SMART theory.

Specific:

Measurable:

Attainable:

Relevant:

Time Bound:

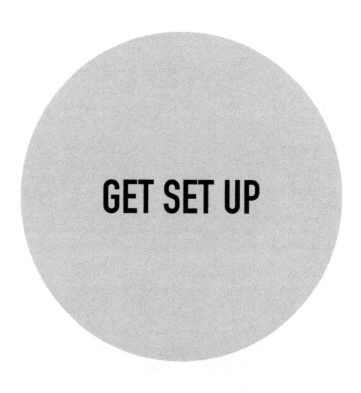

GET SET UP

• Morning Routine •

Get set up for success by crafting your own morning routine.

Here is a sample.

- Get up early
  (eight hours after falling asleep)
- Make my bed
- Drink half a liter of flat water
- Meditate for fifteen minutes

- Write in my *66 Day Journal*
- Review Words of Joy
- Eat breakfast
- Exercise for sixty minutes
- Take a cold shower

Leave your cellphone on airplane mode for the first half of the day and the reactive part of your schedule stops. From now on, others do not have the ability to influence your daily planning.

The day progresses in thirty-minute time slots, which can now be planned by you. Following this plan for the rest of the day protects your decision-making power and sets your productivity on autopilot.

Try it below.

• Evening Routine •

Get set up for success by crafting your own evening routine.

Here is a sample.
- No more caffeine six hours before going to sleep
- No food three hours before going to sleep
- No more screens (TV/phone/tablet/laptop) two hours before going to sleep
- Write in my *66 Day Journal*
- Review Words of Joy
- Read for thirty minutes

Now try it yourself below

_____

_____

_____

_____

_____

_____

_____

_____

_____

_____

_____

_____

• Home Base •

Words of Joy: Tell yourself these words every morning and evening, preferably in the mirror, followed by your goal. In order to find these words, reflect on people, emotions, and situations that made you feel fulfilled and strong. Visualize these situations unfolding in front of you and write these *Words of Joy* from your own precious memories and emotions.

Some examples: Courage, loyalty, openness, strength, clarity, empathy, honesty. Now complete your own list, there is no right or wrong number of words).

_____

_____

_____

_____

_____

_____

_____

_____

My goal: I will...

_____

_____

_____

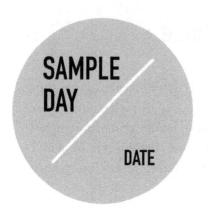

SAMPLE DAY

DATE

Three things I am grateful for (three new things every day)

- MY WARM BED
- MY HEALTH
- THE COOL RAIN, THAT CUTS THROUGH THE STICKY AIR

What am I proud of?

- MY HONESTY DURING THE CONVERSATION I HAD LAST NIGHT
- THAT I GOT UP EARLY TODAY

What am I happy about?

MY HOME, MY ENVIRONMENT, MY CHANCES, MY FREEDOM, THE OPPORTUNITY TO LEARN NEW THINGS

Notes/Thoughts

JOY! WHAT IS THE TITLE OF THE BOOK OF MY LIFE? WHY?
"HAVING" VS. "BEING"
SMILE WITH THE EYES AND THE WHOLE BODY

 Action

Check off your "Big Points" of the morning. What did or didn't you do?

"I haven't failed.
I just found 10,000 ways
That didn't work."
—Thomas Edison

What did I learn today?

HOW GOOD IT FEELS TO PUSH THROUGH A PROJECT, EVEN THOUGH I WAS ALREADY TIRED

What could I have done better?

NOT WATCH TV!

For the next 65 days, I will...

- BE IN THE GYM THREE TIMES PER WEEK
- GO FOR A JOG THREE TIMES PER WEEK

In 65 days, I will...

HAVE LOST FIVE KG

✓ Action

Go back to your home base page
and tell yourself your goal
and your words of joy
in front of the mirror. Enjoy!

3 amazing things that happened today

- TO COME OUT OF THE GYM TIRED, TRULY FEELING PROUD OF MYSELF
- SMILING AT THE CASHIER IN THE SUPERMARKET, AND GETTING A HAPPY SMILE BACK.
- APOLOGIZING HONESTLY TO MY COLLEAGUE AND SEEING HIS JOY AND RELIEF.

The "Big Points" I have to complete today, in order to reach my goal

- 60 MIN IN THE GYM
- 45 MIN JOG
- CREATE A HEALTHY SHOPPING LIST
- WATCH LESS TV
- SMILE MORE
- WRITE IN MY 66 DAY JOURNAL
- TALK OPENLY ABOUT MY GOAL

GET STARTED

• Kick-Off Quarterly Meeting •

Congratulations, let's get started!

Your goal is important! Like in any other successful company, we will have four quarterly meetings in the next 66 days to analyze your performance and to plan the next steps to reach your goal. No worries, there is no dress code!

Olympic gymnasts, world-class athletes, successful entrepreneurs, the biggest pop-stars, and other super performers from different areas all have one thing in common: they visualize the most important parts of what they want to accomplish, *before* they walk out onto the stage.

So, your goal is already a reality, as long as *you* can *see* it.

The likelihood of achieving goals and realizing projects successfully increases exponentially as long as you can visualize the outcome.

✓ Action

Write a letter to yourself describing your 66-day run as if you had already completed it and successfully reached your goal. Write in the second person and talk about all that you have done well and how proud you are of yourself.

• Letter Example •

Dear _____,

It inspires me how disciplined, full of joy, and energetic you have been in knocking out your daily "Big Points." It makes me really proud to see how many people you have inspired with the work you are doing on yourself. It is so wonderful to see you use your time so wisely and get so much more done than before...

On days that are hard, come back, read this letter, and remember the reasons you set out on this unforgettable 66-day journey!
Now, here is some space for your letter, take your time writing it.

• Letter to Self •

Dear _____,

_____

_____

_____

_____

_____

_____

_____

_____

_____

_____

_____

_____

_____

_____

_____

_____

_____

_____

_____

_____

_____

DAY 1

DATE

Three things I am grateful for (three new things every day)

- _____
  _____
- _____
  _____
- _____
  _____

What am I proud of?

_____
_____
_____
_____
_____
_____

What am I happy about?

_____
_____
_____
_____
_____
_____

Notes/Thoughts

_____
_____
_____
_____
_____
_____

✓ Action

Check off your "Big Points" of the morning. What did or didn't you do?

What did I learn today?

_____
_____
_____
_____
_____
_____

*"I haven't failed.
I just found 10,000 ways
that didn't work."*
—Thomas Edison

What could I have done better?

_____
_____
_____
_____
_____
_____
_____

For the next 65 days, I will...

_____
_____
_____
_____
_____
_____
_____

In 65 days, I will...

_____
_____
_____
_____
_____
_____

✓ Action

Go back to your home base
page and tell yourself your goal
and your words of joy
in front of the mirror. Enjoy!

3 amazing things that happened today

• _____
_____
_____

• _____
_____
_____

• _____
_____
_____

The "Big Points" I have to complete today, in order to reach my goal

• _____
_____

• _____
_____

• _____
_____

• _____
_____

• _____
_____

• _____
_____

• _____
_____

DAY 2

DATE

Three things I am grateful for (three new things every day)

- _____
  _____
  _____

- _____
  _____
  _____

- _____
  _____
  _____

What am I proud of?

_____
_____
_____
_____
_____
_____

What am I happy about?

_____
_____
_____
_____
_____
_____

Notes/Thoughts

_____
_____
_____
_____
_____
_____

✓ Action

Check off your "Big Points" of the morning. What did or didn't you do?

"Dance like nobody's watching, love like you've never been hurt, sing like no one's listening, and live like its heaven on earth."
—Mark Twain

What did I learn today?

_____
_____
_____
_____
_____
_____
_____

What could I have done better?

_____
_____
_____
_____
_____
_____
_____

For the next 64 days, I will...

_____
_____
_____
_____
_____
_____

In 64 days, I will...

_____
_____
_____
_____
_____
_____

✅ **Action**

Try eating vegan for a day, just to understand what it feels like

3 amazing things that happened today

- _____
  _____
  _____
- _____
  _____
  _____
- _____
  _____
  _____
  _____

The "Big Points" I have to complete today, in order to reach my goal

- _____
  _____
- _____
  _____
- _____
  _____
- _____
  _____
- _____
  _____
- _____
  _____

DAY 3

DATE

Three things I am grateful for (three new things every day)

- _____
_____

- _____
_____

- _____
_____

What am I proud of?

_____
_____
_____
_____
_____
_____

What am I happy about?

_____
_____
_____
_____
_____

Notes/Thoughts

_____
_____
_____
_____
_____
_____

✓ **Action**

Check off your "Big Points" of the morning. What did or didn't you do?

What did I learn today?

_____
_____
_____
_____
_____
_____
_____

"Because the people who are crazy enough to think they can change the world, are the ones who do."
—Steve Job

What could I have done better?

_____
_____
_____
_____
_____
_____
_____
_____

For the next 63 days, I will...

_____
_____
_____
_____
_____
_____
_____

In 63 days, I will...

_____
_____
_____
_____
_____
_____

✅ Action

Do a seven-minute workout, right now, exactly where you are.

3 amazing things that happened today

- _____
  _____
  _____
- _____
  _____
  _____
- _____
  _____
  _____

The "Big Points" I have to complete today, in order to reach my goal

- _____
- _____
- _____
- _____
- _____
- _____
- _____

DAY 4

DATE

Three things I am grateful for (three new things every day)

- _____
_____

- _____
_____

- _____
_____

What am I proud of?

_____
_____
_____
_____
_____
_____

What am I happy about?

_____
_____
_____
_____
_____
_____

Notes/Thoughts

_____
_____
_____
_____
_____
_____

✓ **Action**

Check off your "Big Points" of the morning. What did or didn't you do?

What did I learn today?

_____
_____
_____
_____
_____
_____

"Success has two letters–
_DO."_
—Johann Wolfgang von Goethe

What could I have done better?

_____
_____
_____
_____
_____
_____
_____

For the next 62 days, I will...

_____
_____
_____
_____
_____
_____
_____

In 62 days, I will...

_____
_____
_____
_____
_____
_____

✅ **Action**

Enjoy the power of silence and meditate for ten minutes today.

3 amazing things that happened today

- _____
_____
_____
- _____
_____
_____
- _____
_____
_____

The "Big Points" I have to complete today, in order to reach my goal

- _____
- _____
- _____
- _____
- _____
- _____
- _____

DAY 5

DATE

**Three things I am grateful for
(three new things every day)**

- _____

- _____

- _____

What am I proud of?

What am I happy about?

Notes/Thoughts

> ✅ **Action**
>
> Check off your "Big Points" of
> the morning. What did or
> didn't you do?

What did I learn today?

> *"It's not bad to fail,
> the only bad thing
> would be not to try."*
> —Heinz Eggert

What could I have done better?

_____
_____
_____
_____
_____
_____
_____
_____

For the next 61 days, I will...

_____
_____
_____
_____
_____
_____

In 61 days, I will...

_____
_____
_____
_____
_____
_____

✅ **Action**

Find an exciting
TED Talk and
watch the video today.

3 amazing things that happened today

- _____
  _____
  _____
- _____
  _____
- _____
  _____
  _____
  _____

The "Big Points" I have to complete today, in order to reach my goal

- _____
  _____
- _____
  _____
- _____
  _____
- _____
  _____
- _____
  _____
- _____
  _____
- _____
  _____

DAY 6

DATE

Three things I am grateful for (three new things every day)

- _____
_____
- _____
_____
- _____
_____

What am I proud of?

_____
_____
_____
_____
_____
_____

What am I happy about?

_____
_____
_____
_____
_____
_____

Notes/Thoughts

_____
_____
_____
_____
_____
_____

✓ Action

Check off your "Big Points" of the morning. What did or didn't you do?

"The best way to predict the future is to create it."
—Willy Brandt

What did I learn today?

_____
_____
_____
_____
_____
_____

What could I have done better?

_____

_____

_____

_____

_____

_____

_____

_____

For the next 60 days, I will...

_____

_____

_____

_____

_____

_____

In 60 days, I will...

_____

_____

_____

_____

_____

_____

Action
Write a card to
a special person today.

3 amazing things that happened today

- _____

_____

_____

- _____

_____

_____

- _____

_____

_____

The "Big Points" I have to complete today, in order to reach my goal

- _____

- _____

- _____

- _____

- _____

- _____

- _____

DAY 7

DATE

Three things I am grateful for (three new things every day)

- _____
  _____

- _____
  _____

- _____
  _____

What am I proud of?

_____
_____
_____
_____
_____
_____

What am I happy about?

_____
_____
_____
_____
_____

Notes/Thoughts

_____
_____
_____
_____
_____
_____

✓ Action

Check off your "Big Points" of the morning. What did or didn't you do?

What did I learn today?

_____
_____
_____
_____
_____
_____
_____

"Success consists of going from failure to failure without loss of enthusiasm."
—Winston Churchill

What could I have done better?

_____

_____

_____

_____

_____

_____

_____

In 59 days, I will...

_____

_____

_____

_____

_____

_____

3 amazing things that happened today

- _____

  _____

  _____

- _____

  _____

  _____

- _____

  _____

  _____

  _____

For the next 59 days, I will...

_____

_____

_____

_____

_____

_____

_____

✅ **Action**

Have the important conversation today, the one that you have been putting off for so long.

The "Big Points" I have to complete today, in order to reach my goal

- _____

  _____

- _____

  _____

- _____

  _____

- _____

  _____

- _____

  _____

- _____

  _____

DAY 8

DATE

Three things I am grateful for (three new things every day)

-
-
-

What am I proud of?

What am I happy about?

Notes/Thoughts

Action

Check off your "Big Points" of the morning. What did or didn't you do?

"Pure insanity is doing the same thing over and over again and expecting different results."
—Albert Einstein

What did I learn today?

What could I have done better?

_____
_____
_____
_____
_____
_____
_____

For the next 58 days, I will...

_____
_____
_____
_____
_____
_____
_____

In 58 days, I will...

_____
_____
_____
_____
_____
_____

✔ **Action**

Talk to a stranger today and have a conversation about the universe.

3 amazing things that happened today

- _____
- _____
- _____

The "Big Points" I have to complete today, in order to reach my goal

- _____
- _____
- _____
- _____
- _____
- _____
- _____

DAY 9

DATE

Three things I am grateful for (three new things every day)

- _____
- _____
- _____

What am I proud of?

What am I happy about?

Notes/Thoughts

✓ **Action**

Check off your "Big Points" of the morning. What did or didn't you do?

What did I learn today?

"Whether you think you can or you think you can't, you're right."
—Henry Ford

What could I have done better?

_____
_____
_____
_____
_____
_____
_____

For the next 57 days, I will...

_____
_____
_____
_____
_____
_____

In 57 days, I will...

_____
_____
_____
_____
_____

✅ Action

Go back to your home base page and tell yourself your goal and your words of joy in front of the mirror. Enjoy!

3 amazing things that happened today

- _____
  _____
  _____
- _____
  _____
  _____
- _____
  _____
  _____

The "Big Points" I have to complete today, in order to reach my goal

- _____
- _____
  _____
- _____
  _____
- _____
  _____
- _____
  _____
- _____
- _____

DAY 10

DATE

Three things I am grateful for (three new things every day)

- _____
- _____
- _____

What am I proud of?

What am I happy about?

Notes/Thoughts

> ✅ **Action**
>
> Check off your "Big Points" of the morning. What did or didn't you do?

What did I learn today?

> *"Do something you're scared of everyday."*
> —Eleanor Roosevelt

What could I have done better?

_____
_____
_____
_____
_____
_____
_____

For the next 56 days, I will...

_____
_____
_____
_____
_____
_____

In 56 days, I will...

_____
_____
_____
_____
_____
_____

> ✔ **Action**
>
> Try going without caffeine, nicotine, alcohol, and sugar today.

3 amazing things that happened today

- _____
  _____
  _____

- _____
  _____
  _____

- _____
  _____
  _____

The "Big Points" I have to complete today, in order to reach my goal

- _____
- _____
  _____
- _____
  _____
- _____
  _____
- _____
  _____
- _____
  _____

DAY 11

DATE

Three things I am grateful for (three new things every day)

- _____
_____
_____

- _____
_____
_____

- _____
_____

What am I proud of?

_____
_____
_____
_____
_____
_____
_____

What am I happy about?

_____
_____
_____
_____
_____
_____
_____

Notes/Thoughts

_____
_____
_____
_____
_____
_____

Action

Check off your "Big Points" of the morning. What did or didn't you do?

What did I learn today?

_____
_____
_____
_____
_____
_____
_____

"Only he who burns, can spark a fire."
—Augustinus Aurelius

What could I have done better?

_____
_____
_____
_____
_____
_____
_____
_____

In 55 days, I will...

_____
_____
_____
_____
_____
_____

3 amazing things that happened today

- _____
_____
_____
- _____
_____
_____
- _____
_____
_____

For the next 55 days, I will...

_____
_____
_____
_____
_____
_____

✓ **Action**

Print out an interesting Wikipedia article, study it, and tell someone today about what you learned.

The "Big Points" I have to complete today, in order to reach my goal

- _____
- _____
- _____
- _____
- _____
- _____

DAY 12

DATE

Three things I am grateful for (three new things every day)

- _____
- _____
- _____

What am I proud of?

What am I happy about?

Notes/Thoughts

✓ Action

Check off your "Big Points" of the morning. What did or didn't you do?

What did I learn today?

"The one who wants it, will find ways, the one who doesn't want it, will find reasons."
—Götz Werner

What could I have done better?

_____
_____
_____
_____
_____
_____
_____
_____

For the next 54 days, I will...

_____
_____
_____
_____
_____
_____
_____

In 54 days, I will...

_____
_____
_____
_____
_____
_____

✔ Action

Get up at five tomorrow and
enjoy the sunrise
and the silence.

3 amazing things that happened today

- _____
  _____
  _____
- _____
  _____
  _____
- _____
  _____
  _____

The "Big Points" I have to complete today, in order to reach my goal

- _____
  _____
- _____
  _____
- _____
  _____
- _____
  _____
- _____
  _____
- _____
  _____

DAY 13

DATE

Three things I am grateful for (three new things every day)

- _____
  _____

- _____
  _____

- _____
  _____

What am I proud of?

_____
_____
_____
_____
_____
_____

What am I happy about?

_____
_____
_____
_____
_____

Notes/Thoughts

_____
_____
_____
_____
_____
_____

✅ Action

Check off your "Big Points" of the morning. What did or didn't you do?

What did I learn today?

_____
_____
_____
_____
_____
_____

"The one who follows the footsteps of somebody else, will not leave his own tracks."
—Wilhelm Busch

**What could I have
done better?**

_____
_____
_____
_____
_____
_____
_____

**For the next 53 days,
I will...**

_____
_____
_____
_____
_____
_____
_____

In 53 days, I will...

_____
_____
_____
_____
_____
_____

✅ Action

Take an ice cold shower and see
how you feel afterwards.

**3 amazing things that
happened today**

- _____
  _____
  _____
- _____
  _____
  _____
- _____
  _____
  _____
  _____

**The "Big Points" I have to
complete today, in order to
reach my goal**

- _____
  _____
- _____
  _____
- _____
  _____
- _____
  _____
- _____
  _____
- _____
  _____
- _____
  _____

DAY 14

/

DATE

Three things I am grateful for (three new things every day)

- _____
  _____

- _____
  _____

- _____
  _____

What am I proud of?

_____
_____
_____
_____
_____
_____
_____

What am I happy about?

_____
_____
_____
_____
_____
_____
_____

Notes/Thoughts

_____
_____
_____
_____
_____
_____

✅ **Action**

Check off your "Big Points" of the morning. What did or didn't you do?

What did I learn today?

_____
_____
_____
_____
_____
_____
_____
_____

"If you do what you've always done, you'll get what you've always gotten."
—Anthony Robbins

**What could I have
done better?**

_____

_____

_____

_____

_____

_____

_____

**For the next 52 days,
I will...**

_____

_____

_____

_____

_____

_____

In 52 days, I will...

_____

_____

_____

_____

_____

_____

> ✅ **Action**
>
> "Survive" an entire day with your
> phone in airplane mode.

**3 amazing things that
happened today**

- _____

_____

_____

- _____

_____

_____

- _____

_____

_____

**The "Big Points" I have to
complete today, in order to
reach my goal**

- _____

_____

- _____

_____

- _____

_____

- _____

_____

- _____

_____

- _____

_____

DAY 15

DATE

Three things I am grateful for (three new things every day)

- _____
- _____
- _____

What am I proud of?

What am I happy about?

Notes/Thoughts

> ✅ **Action**
>
> Check off your "Big Points" of the morning. What did or didn't you do?

What did I learn today?

> *"Don't think too much about what you don't have but what you do have."*
> —Marc Aurel

What could I have done better?

_____
_____
_____
_____
_____
_____
_____

In 51 days, I will...

_____
_____
_____
_____
_____
_____

3 amazing things that happened today

- _____
  _____
  _____
- _____
  _____
  _____
- _____
  _____
  _____

For the next 51 days, I will...

_____
_____
_____
_____
_____
_____
_____

✓ **Action**

What did you love doing as a kid? That is exactly what you will do tomorrow.

The "Big Points" I have to complete today, in order to reach my goal

- _____
  _____
- _____
  _____
- _____
  _____
- _____
  _____
- _____
  _____
- _____
  _____
- _____

DAY 16

DATE

Three things I am grateful for (three new things every day)

- _____
- _____
- _____

What am I proud of?

What am I happy about?

Notes/Thoughts

> ✓ **Action**
>
> Check off your "Big Points" of the morning. What did or didn't you do?

What did I learn today?

> *"Only those who dare to fail greatly can ever achieve greatly."*
> —Robert F. Kennedy

**What could I have
done better?**

_____

_____

_____

_____

_____

_____

_____

_____

**For the next 50 days,
I will...**

_____

_____

_____

_____

_____

_____

_____

In 50 days, I will...

_____

_____

_____

_____

_____

_____

✓ **Action**

Borrow a skateboard and ask
a skateboarder to show you
how to kickflip.

**3 amazing things that
happened today**

- _____

  _____

  _____

- _____

  _____

  _____

- _____

  _____

  _____

**The "Big Points" I have to
complete today, in order to
reach my goal**

- _____

  _____

- _____

  _____

- _____

  _____

- _____

  _____

- _____

  _____

- _____

  _____

First Quarterly Meeting

Congratulations, you have reached 25 percent of your goal!

During the last sixteen days, you've gone through a variety of day-to-day activities, and you can now begin to understand the basis of your most successful and fulfilling days. We will continue to build upon this structure as we focus on the variables that work to develop "your best day."

Regarding the continuous implementation of this exact daily structure, you will create a VISION AGREEMENT—a contract you make with yourself.

 Action

Write down the structure of your "best day." What has to happen so that you end the day proud, happy, and truly fulfilled?

Vision Agreement

My Best Day

_____

_____

_____

_____

_____

_____

_____

_____

_____

_____

_____

_____

_____

I hereby confirm that the above-mentioned daily structure enable the realization of my goal in the best way possible. If I continue to implement this daily routine for the next fifty days, I will reach my goal. As the above-mentioned daily routine also makes me proud and happy, I hereby declare to live the following fifty days according to this plan and as my "best days."

_____

Place, Date, Signature

DAY 17

DATE

Three things I am grateful for (three new things every day)

- _____

- _____

- _____

What am I proud of?

What am I happy about?

Notes/Thoughts

> **✓ Action**
>
> Check off your "Big Points" of the morning. What did or didn't you do?

What did I learn today?

> _"Dissatisfaction is the first step to success."_
> —Oscar Wilde

What could I have done better?

_____
_____
_____
_____
_____
_____
_____

In 49 days, I will...

_____
_____
_____
_____
_____

3 amazing things that happened today

- _____
  _____
  _____
- _____
  _____
  _____
- _____
  _____
  _____

For the next 49 days, I will...

_____
_____
_____
_____
_____
_____
_____

✔ Action

Go back to your home base page and tell yourself your goal and your words of joy in front of the mirror. Enjoy!

The "Big Points" I have to complete today, in order to reach my goal

- _____
- _____
- _____
- _____
- _____
- _____
- _____

DAY 18

DATE

Three things I am grateful for (three new things every day)

- _____
  _____

- _____
  _____

- _____
  _____

What am I proud of?

_____
_____
_____
_____
_____
_____

What am I happy about?

_____
_____
_____
_____
_____
_____

Notes/Thoughts

_____
_____
_____
_____
_____
_____

✓ **Action**

Check off your "Big Points" of the morning. What did or didn't you do?

"To fail is a detour, not a dead-end street."
—Zig Ziglar

What did I learn today?

_____
_____
_____
_____
_____
_____
_____

What could I have done better?

_____
_____
_____
_____
_____
_____
_____
_____

For the next 48 days, I will...

_____
_____
_____
_____
_____
_____
_____

In 48 days, I will...

_____
_____
_____
_____
_____
_____

✓ Action

Find a basketball court and hit a three-point shot

3 amazing things that happened today

- _____
  _____
  _____
- _____
  _____
  _____
- _____
  _____
  _____

The "Big Points" I have to complete today, in order to reach my goal

- _____
- _____
- _____
- _____
- _____
- _____
- _____

DAY 19

DATE

Three things I am grateful for (three new things every day)

- _____
  _____
  _____

- _____
  _____
  _____

- _____
  _____

What am I proud of?

_____
_____
_____
_____
_____
_____
_____

What am I happy about?

_____
_____
_____
_____
_____
_____

Notes/Thoughts

_____
_____
_____
_____
_____
_____

✔ **Action**

Check off your "Big Points" of the morning. What did or didn't you do?

What did I learn today?

_____
_____
_____
_____
_____
_____
_____

"Hard work doesn't guarantee success, but increases its chances."
—B. J. Gupta

What could I have done better?

_____
_____
_____
_____
_____
_____
_____
_____

In 47 days, I will...

_____
_____
_____
_____
_____
_____

3 amazing things that happened today

- _____
_____
_____
- _____
_____
- _____
_____
_____

For the next 47 days, I will...

_____
_____
_____
_____
_____
_____

✓ **Action**

Before you go to bed today, go for a walk and kiss the ground with every step. If possible, walk barefoot and feel the grass, snow or sand.

The "Big Points" I have to complete today, in order to reach my goal

- _____
_____
- _____
_____
- _____
_____
- _____
_____
- _____
_____
- _____
_____

DAY 20

DATE

Three things I am grateful for (three new things every day)

- _____
  _____

- _____
  _____

- _____
  _____

What am I proud of?

_____
_____
_____
_____
_____
_____

What am I happy about?

_____
_____
_____
_____
_____
_____

Notes/Thoughts

_____
_____
_____
_____
_____
_____

✔ **Action**

Check off your "Big Points" of the morning. What did or didn't you do?

What did I learn today?

_____
_____
_____
_____
_____
_____

"You must expect great things of yourself before you can do them."
—Michael Jordan

**What could I have
done better?**

_____

_____

_____

_____

_____

_____

_____

**For the next 46 days,
I will...**

_____

_____

_____

_____

_____

_____

In 46 days, I will...

_____

_____

_____

_____

_____

_____

✅ **Action**

Go to the window and take ten deep
breaths (in through the nose, out
through the mouth).

**3 amazing things that
happened today**

- _____

_____

_____

- _____

_____

_____

- _____

_____

_____

**The "Big Points" I have to
complete today, in order to
reach my goal**

- _____

- _____

- _____

- _____

- _____

- _____

- _____

DAY 21

DATE

Three things I am grateful for (three new things every day)

- _____
- _____
- _____

What am I proud of?

What am I happy about?

Notes/Thoughts

✓ Action

Check off your "Big Points" of the morning. What did or didn't you do?

What did I learn today?

"Paths are made by walking."
—Franz Kafka

**What could I have
done better?**

_____

_____

_____

_____

_____

_____

_____

**For the next 45 days,
I will...**

_____

_____

_____

_____

_____

_____

_____

In 45 days, I will...

_____

_____

_____

_____

_____

_____

✅ **Action**

Read in an inspiring book
for ten minutes
before you fall asleep.

**3 amazing things that
happened today**

- _____

  _____

  _____

- _____

  _____

  _____

- _____

  _____

  _____

**The "Big Points" I have to
complete today, in order to
reach my goal**

- _____

- _____

- _____

- _____

- _____

- _____

- _____

DAY 22

DATE

**Three things I am grateful for
(three new things every day)**

- _____
  _____

- _____
  _____

- _____
  _____

What am I proud of?

_____
_____
_____
_____
_____
_____

What am I happy about?

_____
_____
_____
_____
_____

Notes/Thoughts

_____
_____
_____
_____
_____
_____

✔ **Action**

Check off your "Big Points" of
the morning. What did or
didn't you do?

What did I learn today?

_____
_____
_____
_____
_____
_____
_____

_"If your dreams don't scare you,
they are not big enough."_
—Ellen Johnson-Sirleaf

What could I have done better?

_____
_____
_____
_____
_____
_____
_____
_____

For the next 44 days, I will...

_____
_____
_____
_____
_____
_____
_____

In 44 days, I will...

_____
_____
_____
_____
_____
_____

✓ Action

Call an old friend today, and ask about how they are.

3 amazing things that happened today

- _____
_____
_____
- _____
_____
_____
- _____
_____
_____
_____

The "Big Points" I have to complete today, in order to reach my goal

- _____
- _____
- _____
- _____
- _____
- _____
- _____

DAY 23

DATE

Three things I am grateful for (three new things every day)

- _____
- _____
- _____

What am I proud of?

What am I happy about?

Notes/Thoughts

✔ **Action**

Check off your "Big Points" of the morning. What did or didn't you do?

What did I learn today?

"Life begins at the end of your comfort zone."
—Neale Donald Walsch

What could I have done better?

_____

_____

_____

_____

_____

_____

_____

_____

In 43 days, I will...

_____

_____

_____

_____

_____

_____

3 amazing things that happened today

• _____

_____

_____

• _____

_____

_____

• _____

_____

_____

_____

For the next 43 days, I will...

_____

_____

_____

_____

_____

_____

✅ **Action**

After waking up,
stay in bed and smile at
the ceiling for three minutes.

The "Big Points" I have to complete today, in order to reach my goal

• _____

• _____

• _____

• _____

• _____

• _____

• _____

DAY 24

DATE

Three things I am grateful for (three new things every day)

- _____
- _____
- _____

What am I proud of?

What am I happy about?

Notes/Thoughts

✅ Action

Check off your "Big Points" of the morning. What did or didn't you do?

What did I learn today?

"Change your thoughts and you change your world."
—Norman Vincent Peale

What could I have done better?

_____
_____
_____
_____
_____
_____
_____

For the next 42 days, I will...

_____
_____
_____
_____
_____
_____
_____

In 42 days, I will...

_____
_____
_____
_____
_____
_____

✓ **Action**

Go without Playstation, Youtube, gaming apps, or TV today.

3 amazing things that happened today

- _____
  _____
- _____
  _____
- _____
  _____

The "Big Points" I have to complete today, in order to reach my goal

- _____
- _____
- _____
- _____
- _____
- _____

DAY 25

DATE

Three things I am grateful for (three new things every day)

-
-
-

What am I proud of?

What am I happy about?

Notes/Thoughts

Action

Check off your "Big Points" of the morning. What did or didn't you do?

"The only true test of values, either of men or of things, is that of their ability to make the world a better place in which to live."
—Henry Ford

What did I learn today?

What could I have done better?

_____
_____
_____
_____
_____
_____
_____
_____

For the next 41 days, I will...

_____
_____
_____
_____
_____
_____

In 41 days, I will...

_____
_____
_____
_____
_____
_____

✓ Action

Go back to your home base
page and tell yourself your goal
and your words of joy
in front of the mirror. Enjoy!

3 amazing things that happened today

- _____
  _____
  _____
- _____
  _____
  _____
- _____
  _____
  _____

The "Big Points" I have to complete today, in order to reach my goal

- _____
- _____
  _____
- _____
- _____
- _____
- _____
- _____

DAY 26

DATE

**Three things I am grateful for
(three new things every day)**

- _____

- _____

- _____

What am I proud of?

_____
_____
_____
_____
_____
_____

What am I happy about?

_____
_____
_____
_____
_____
_____

Notes/Thoughts

_____
_____
_____
_____
_____
_____

✅ **Action**

Check off your "Big Points" of
the morning. What did or
didn't you do?

What did I learn today?

_____
_____
_____
_____
_____
_____

_"Most people die at 25 but are
buried at 75."_
—Benjamin Franklin

What could I have done better?

_____
_____
_____
_____
_____
_____
_____

For the next 40 days, I will...

_____
_____
_____
_____
_____
_____
_____

In 40 days, I will...

_____
_____
_____
_____
_____
_____

✓ Action

Surprise a special person today with something small you cooked or baked yourself.

3 amazing things that happened today

- _____
  _____
  _____
- _____
  _____
  _____
- _____
  _____
  _____
  _____

The "Big Points" I have to complete today, in order to reach my goal

- _____
  _____
- _____
  _____
- _____
  _____
- _____
  _____
- _____
  _____
- _____
  _____

DAY 27

DATE

Three things I am grateful for (three new things every day)

- _____
- _____
- _____

What am I proud of?

What am I happy about?

Notes/Thoughts

✓ **Action**

Check off your "Big Points" of the morning. What did or didn't you do?

What did I learn today?

"We cannot solve our problems with the same thinking we used when we created them."
—Albert Einstein

What could I have done better?

_____
_____
_____
_____
_____
_____
_____

For the next 39 days, I will...

_____
_____
_____
_____
_____
_____
_____

In 39 days, I will...

_____
_____
_____
_____
_____
_____

✅ Action

Take a different way home today and learn about new parts of your area.

3 amazing things that happened today

- _____
_____
_____
- _____
_____
_____
- _____
_____
_____

The "Big Points" I have to complete today, in order to reach my goal

- _____
_____
- _____
_____
- _____
_____
- _____
_____
- _____
_____
- _____
_____

DAY 28

DATE

**Three things I am grateful for
(three new things every day)**

- _____
_____
- _____
_____
- _____
_____

What am I proud of?

_____
_____
_____
_____
_____
_____

What am I happy about?

_____
_____
_____
_____
_____

Notes/Thoughts

_____
_____
_____
_____
_____
_____

✓ **Action**

Check off your "Big Points" of
the morning. What did or
didn't you do?

What did I learn today?

_____
_____
_____
_____
_____
_____
_____

*The biggest mistake one can
ever make is to always fear
to make a mistake."*
—Dietrich Bonhoeffer

What could I have done better?

_____
_____
_____
_____
_____
_____
_____
_____

For the next 38 days, I will...

_____
_____
_____
_____
_____
_____

In 38 days, I will...

_____
_____
_____
_____
_____
_____

✅ **Action**

Buy movie tickets
and go to see a comedy with
someone special today.

3 amazing things that happened today

- _____
  _____
  _____
- _____
  _____
- _____
  _____
  _____

The "Big Points" I have to complete today, in order to reach my goal

- _____
- _____
- _____
- _____
- _____
- _____
- _____

DAY 29

DATE

Three things I am grateful for (three new things every day)

- _____

- _____

- _____

What am I proud of?

What am I happy about?

Notes/Thoughts

✅ **Action**

Check off your "Big Points" of the morning. What did or didn't you do?

What did I learn today?

"A person with a new idea is called crazy until the idea succeeds."
—Mark Twain

**What could I have
done better?**

_____
_____
_____
_____
_____
_____
_____

**For the next 37 days,
I will...**

_____
_____
_____
_____
_____
_____

In 37 days, I will...

_____
_____
_____
_____
_____

✅ **Action**

Smile at
a stranger today.

**3 amazing things that
happened today**

- _____
_____
_____
- _____
_____
_____
- _____
_____
_____

**The "Big Points" I have to
complete today, in order to
reach my goal**

- _____
- _____
- _____
- _____
- _____
- _____
- _____

DAY 30

DATE

Three things I am grateful for (three new things every day)

- _____
- _____
- _____

What am I proud of?

_____
_____
_____
_____
_____
_____

What am I happy about?

_____
_____
_____
_____
_____

Notes/Thoughts

_____
_____
_____
_____
_____
_____

✓ **Action**

Check off your "Big Points" of the morning. What did or didn't you do?

What did I learn today?

_____
_____
_____
_____
_____
_____

"You have to do what few people do, to have what few people have."
—Les Brown

What could I have done better?

_____

_____

_____

_____

_____

_____

_____

For the next 36 days, I will...

_____

_____

_____

_____

_____

_____

In 36 days, I will...

_____

_____

_____

_____

_____

✓ Action

Drink three liters
of flat water today.

3 amazing things that happened today

- _____

  _____

- _____

  _____

- _____

  _____

The "Big Points" I have to complete today, in order to reach my goal

- _____

- _____

- _____

- _____

- _____

- _____

DAY 31

DATE

Three things I am grateful for (three new things every day)

- _____
- _____
- _____

What am I proud of?

What am I happy about?

Notes/Thoughts

✓ Action

Check off your "Big Points" of the morning. What did or didn't you do?

"You have to attempt the impossible to achieve the possible."
—Hermann Hesse

What did I learn today?

What could I have done better?

_____
_____
_____
_____
_____
_____
_____
_____

For the next 35 days, I will...

_____
_____
_____
_____
_____
_____
_____
_____

In 35 days, I will...

_____
_____
_____
_____
_____
_____
_____

✅ **Action**

Apologize to someone today.

3 amazing things that happened today

- _____
_____
_____
- _____
_____
_____
- _____
_____
_____

The "Big Points" I have to complete today, in order to reach my goal

- _____
_____
- _____
_____
- _____
_____
- _____
_____
- _____
_____
- _____
_____

DAY 32

DATE

Three things I am grateful for (three new things every day)

- _____
- _____
- _____

What am I proud of?

What am I happy about?

Notes/Thoughts

> ✓ **Action**
>
> Check off your "Big Points" of the morning. What did or didn't you do?

What did I learn today?

"Choose a job you love and you don't have to work for the rest of your life."
—Confucius

What could I have done better?

_____
_____
_____
_____
_____
_____
_____
_____

For the next 34 days, I will...

_____
_____
_____
_____
_____
_____
_____

In 34 days, I will...

_____
_____
_____
_____
_____

✓ Action

Ask an older person about an important life lesson today.

3 amazing things that happened today

- _____
_____
_____
- _____
_____
_____
- _____
_____
_____

The "Big Points" I have to complete today, in order to reach my goal

- _____
- _____
- _____
- _____
- _____
- _____
- _____

DAY 33

DATE

Three things I am grateful for (three new things every day)

- _____
  _____
  _____

- _____
  _____
  _____

- _____
  _____
  _____

What am I proud of?

_____
_____
_____
_____
_____
_____
_____

What am I happy about?

_____
_____
_____
_____
_____
_____
_____

Notes/Thoughts

_____
_____
_____
_____
_____
_____

✓ Action

Check off your "Big Points" of the morning. What did or didn't you do?

"Constancy is the complement of all other human virtues."
—Giuseppe Mazzini

What did I learn today?

_____
_____
_____
_____
_____
_____
_____

What could I have done better?

_____
_____
_____
_____
_____
_____
_____

In 33 days, I will...

_____
_____
_____
_____
_____

3 amazing things that happened today

- _____
  _____
  _____
- _____
  _____
  _____
- _____
  _____
  _____

For the next 33 days, I will...

_____
_____
_____
_____
_____
_____
_____

✔ Action

Go back to your home base page and tell yourself your goal and your words of joy in front of the mirror. Enjoy!

The "Big Points" I have to complete today, in order to reach my goal

- _____
  _____
- _____
  _____
- _____
  _____
- _____
  _____
- _____
  _____
- _____

Quarterly Meeting 2

Congratulations, you have reached 50 percent of your goal!

While you are reading these words, you already belong to the few people who keep pushing until half-time and don't give up after just a few weeks. Be proud of yourself and take a look back over your shoulder, at all your hard work, to understand how far you have come.

Action I

New places have the ability to break old patterns and create new energy. If you usually write in your *66 Day Journal* in the same place (e.g. your desk), look for a new place today where you will hold this quarterly meeting. Today, maybe try the garden, the balcony, on the floor, or a quiet café? New paths always create new perspectives.

Action II

Turn back the pages and take a look at the past days, and all the "Big Points" you hit on your journey to your goal—enjoy the feeling, it's true fulfillment! You have accomplished a lot!

What important things did I implement in the last thirty-three days?

_____

_____

_____

_____

_____

_____

_____

_____

What can I improve in the next thirty-three days?

_____

_____

_____

_____

_____

_____

_____

_____

_____

TRUST

In our pursuit of great goals, fear, doubt, confusion, and uncertainty can always enter our thinking. It's the same for everyone and completely normal. A very effective way to accept and transmute these internal obstacles is the ability to identify them. Identify your limiting thoughts, and they become powerless.

Like a feather that gently touches a glass, know and feel exactly what voice is speaking inside of you. "Ah, this is insecurity," or "OK, that is fear." Don't go too fast; it's not a guessing-game, just an opportunity to calm your mind. Allow your thoughts to move like a drop of water in a river, or like clouds in the sky. Always know, behind every cloud is a clear, blue sky. You are not the wave; you are the ocean!

Continued joy and fulfillment for the next thirty-three days!

I am especially proud of...

_____

DAY 34

DATE

Three things I am grateful for (three new things every day)

- _____
- _____
- _____

What am I proud of?

What am I happy about?

Notes/Thoughts

✅ **Action**

Check off your "Big Points" of the morning. What did or didn't you do?

What did I learn today?

"He who fights, may lose.
He who doesn't fight has already lost."
—Bertolt Brecht

What could I have done better?

_____

_____

_____

_____

_____

_____

_____

For the next 32 days, I will...

_____

_____

_____

_____

_____

_____

In 32 days, I will...

_____

_____

_____

_____

_____

_____

✓ **Action**

Do a seven-minute workout, right now, exactly where you are.

3 amazing things that happened today

- _____

_____

_____

- _____

_____

_____

- _____

_____

_____

The "Big Points" I have to complete today, in order to reach my goal

- _____

_____

- _____

- _____

_____

- _____

- _____

_____

- _____

DAY 35

DATE

Three things I am grateful for (three new things every day)

- _____
  _____
  _____

- _____
  _____
  _____

- _____
  _____

What am I proud of?

_____
_____
_____
_____
_____
_____
_____

What am I happy about?

_____
_____
_____
_____
_____
_____
_____

Notes/Thoughts

_____
_____
_____
_____
_____
_____
_____

✅ **Action**

Check off your "Big Points" of the morning. What did or didn't you do?

What did I learn today?

_____
_____
_____
_____
_____
_____
_____

"What great thing would you attempt if you knew you could not fail?"
—Robert H. Schuller

**What could I have
done better?**

_____
_____
_____
_____
_____
_____
_____

**For the next 31 days,
I will...**

_____
_____
_____
_____
_____
_____

In 31 days, I will...

_____
_____
_____
_____
_____
_____

✅ **Action**

Enjoy the power of silence and
meditate for ten minutes today.

**3 amazing things that
happened today**

- _____
  _____
  _____
- _____
  _____
- _____
  _____
  _____

**The "Big Points" I have to
complete today, in order to
reach my goal**

- _____
- _____
- _____
- _____
- _____
- _____
- _____

DAY 36

DATE

Three things I am grateful for (three new things every day)

- _____
  _____
- _____
  _____
- _____
  _____

What am I proud of?

_____
_____
_____
_____
_____
_____
_____

What am I happy about?

_____
_____
_____
_____
_____
_____

Notes/Thoughts

_____
_____
_____
_____
_____
_____
_____

Action

Check off your "Big Points" of the morning. What did or didn't you do?

What did I learn today?

_____
_____
_____
_____
_____
_____
_____

"A winner is a dreamer who never gives up."
—Nelson Mandela

What could I have done better?

_____
_____
_____
_____
_____
_____
_____
_____

For the next 30 days, I will...

_____
_____
_____
_____
_____
_____
_____

In 30 days, I will...

_____
_____
_____
_____
_____
_____

✓ Action

Find another exciting TED Talk and watch the video today.

3 amazing things that happened today

- _____
  _____
  _____
- _____
  _____
  _____
- _____
  _____
  _____
  _____

The "Big Points" I have to complete today, in order to reach my goal

- _____
  _____
- _____
  _____
- _____
  _____
- _____
  _____
- _____
  _____
- _____
  _____
- _____
  _____

DAY 37

DATE

Three things I am grateful for (three new things every day)

- _____
  _____

- _____
  _____

- _____
  _____

What am I proud of?

_____
_____
_____
_____
_____
_____

What am I happy about?

_____
_____
_____
_____
_____
_____

Notes/Thoughts

_____
_____
_____
_____
_____
_____

✅ **Action**

Check off your "Big Points" of the morning. What did or didn't you do?

What did I learn today?

_____
_____
_____
_____
_____
_____
_____

"We must use time as a tool, not as a couch."
—John F. Kennedy

**What could I have
done better?**

_____
_____
_____
_____
_____
_____
_____

**For the next 29 days,
I will...**

_____
_____
_____
_____
_____
_____

In 29 days, I will...

_____
_____
_____
_____
_____

✅ **Action**

Write a card
to a special person today.

**3 amazing things that
happened today**

- _____
  _____
  _____
- _____
  _____
  _____
- _____
  _____
  _____

**The "Big Points" I have to
complete today, in order to
reach my goal**

- _____
- _____
- _____
- _____
- _____
- _____
- _____

DAY 38

DATE

Three things I am grateful for (three new things every day)

- _____
  _____
  _____

- _____
  _____
  _____

- _____
  _____
  _____

What am I proud of?

_____
_____
_____
_____
_____
_____
_____

What am I happy about?

_____
_____
_____
_____
_____
_____
_____

Notes/Thoughts

_____
_____
_____
_____
_____
_____

✅ **Action**

Check off your "Big Points" of the morning. What did or didn't you do?

"The true secret to success is enthusiasm."
—Walter Chrysler

What did I learn today?

_____
_____
_____
_____
_____
_____
_____
_____

**What could I have
done better?**

_____

_____

_____

_____

_____

_____

_____

**For the next 28 days,
I will...**

_____

_____

_____

_____

_____

_____

_____

In 28 days, I will...

_____

_____

_____

_____

_____

_____

✅ **Action**

Have an important conversation
today that you have been
putting off for so long.

**3 amazing things that
happened today**

- _____

  _____

  _____

- _____

  _____

- _____

  _____

  _____

**The "Big Points" I have to
complete today, in order to
reach my goal**

- _____

  _____

- _____

  _____

- _____

  _____

- _____

  _____

- _____

  _____

- _____

  _____

- _____

  _____

DAY 39

/

DATE

Three things I am grateful for (three new things every day)

- _____

- _____

- _____

What am I proud of?

_____
_____
_____
_____
_____
_____
_____

What am I happy about?

_____
_____
_____
_____
_____
_____
_____

Notes/Thoughts

_____
_____
_____
_____
_____
_____

✓ Action

Check off your "Big Points" of the morning. What did or didn't you do?

What did I learn today?

_____
_____
_____
_____
_____
_____

> "It's not that we have little time,
> but more that we waste
> a good deal of it."
> —Lucius Annaeus Seneca

What could I have done better?

_____

_____

_____

_____

_____

_____

_____

For the next 27 days, I will...

_____

_____

_____

_____

_____

_____

In 27 days, I will...

_____

_____

_____

_____

_____

_____

✅ **Action**

Try eating vegan for another day.
How does it feel?

3 amazing things that happened today

- _____

  _____

  _____

- _____

  _____

  _____

- _____

  _____

  _____

The "Big Points" I have to complete today, in order to reach my goal

- _____

- _____

- _____

- _____

- _____

- _____

- _____

DAY 40

DATE

Three things I am grateful for (three new things every day)

- _____
_____

- _____
_____

- _____
_____

What am I proud of?

What am I happy about?

Notes/Thoughts

> ✓ **Action**
>
> Check off your "Big Points" of the morning. What did or didn't you do?

What did I learn today?

"Kindness is a language that can be heard by the deaf and read by the blind."
—Mark Twain

What could I have done better?

_____

_____

_____

_____

_____

_____

_____

For the next 26 days, I will...

_____

_____

_____

_____

_____

_____

In 26 days, I will...

_____

_____

_____

_____

_____

✅ **Action**

Talk to a stranger today and have a conversation about the universe.

3 amazing things that happened today

- _____

  _____

  _____

- _____

  _____

  _____

- _____

  _____

  _____

The "Big Points" I have to complete today, in order to reach my goal

- _____

  _____

- _____

  _____

- _____

  _____

- _____

  _____

- _____

  _____

- _____

  _____

- _____

DAY 41

DATE

Three things I am grateful for (three new things every day)

- _____
  _____
  _____

- _____
  _____
  _____

- _____
  _____

What am I proud of?

_____
_____
_____
_____
_____
_____

What am I happy about?

_____
_____
_____
_____
_____
_____

Notes/Thoughts

_____
_____
_____
_____
_____
_____

✓ **Action**

Check off your "Big Points" of the morning. What did or didn't you do?

"Obstacles are things that a man sees when he takes his eye off the goal."
—E. Joseph Cossman

What did I learn today?

_____
_____
_____
_____
_____
_____
_____

What could I have done better?

_____
_____
_____
_____
_____
_____
_____
_____

For the next 25 days, I will...

_____
_____
_____
_____
_____
_____

In 25 days, I will...

_____
_____
_____
_____
_____
_____

✓ **Action**

Go back to your home base
page and tell yourself your goal
and your words of joy
in front of the mirror. Enjoy!

3 amazing things that happened today

• _____
_____
_____
• _____
_____
_____
• _____
_____
_____

The "Big Points" I have to complete today, in order to reach my goal

• _____
• _____
• _____
• _____
• _____
• _____
• _____

DAY 42

DATE

Three things I am grateful for (three new things every day)

- _____
- _____
- _____

What am I proud of?

What am I happy about?

Notes/Thoughts

✓ **Action**

Check off your "Big Points" of the morning. What did or didn't you do?

What did I learn today?

"Money isn't something I play for. I want to compete. I want to win."
—Dirk Nowitzki

**What could I have
done better?**

_____
_____
_____
_____
_____
_____
_____
_____

**For the next 24 days,
I will...**

_____
_____
_____
_____
_____
_____
_____

In 24 days, I will...

_____
_____
_____
_____
_____
_____

> ✔ **Action**
>
> Try going without caffeine,
> nicotine, alcohol,
> or sugar today.

**3 amazing things that
happened today**

- _____
  _____
  _____
- _____
  _____
  _____
- _____
  _____
  _____

**The "Big Points" I have to
complete today, in order to
reach my goal**

- _____
- _____
- _____
- _____
- _____
- _____
- _____

DAY 43

DATE

Three things I am grateful for (three new things every day)

- _____
- _____
- _____

What am I proud of?

What am I happy about?

Notes/Thoughts

✅ Action

Check off your "Big Points" of the morning. What did or didn't you do?

What did I learn today?

"You don't have to be great to begin, but you have to begin to be great."
—Zig Ziglar

What could I have done better?

_____

_____

_____

_____

_____

_____

_____

For the next 23 days, I will...

_____

_____

_____

_____

_____

_____

_____

In 23 days, I will...

_____

_____

_____

_____

_____

✔ Action

Print out an interesting Wikipedia article, study it, and tell someone today about what you learned.

3 amazing things that happened today

- _____

  _____

  _____

- _____

  _____

  _____

- _____

  _____

  _____

  _____

The "Big Points" I have to complete today, in order to reach my goal

- _____

- _____

  _____

- _____

- _____

- _____

- _____

- _____

DAY 44

DATE

Three things I am grateful for (three new things every day)

-
-
-

What am I proud of?

What am I happy about?

Notes/Thoughts

✅ **Action**

Check off your "Big Points" of the morning. What did or didn't you do?

What did I learn today?

"You are the average of the five people you spend the most time with."
—Jim Rohn

**What could I have
done better?**

_____

_____

_____

_____

_____

_____

_____

_____

**For the next 22 days,
I will...**

_____

_____

_____

_____

_____

_____

_____

In 22 days, I will...

_____

_____

_____

_____

_____

_____

✅ **Action**

Get up at five tomorrow and
enjoy the sunrise and the silence.

**3 amazing things that
happened today**

- _____

_____

_____

- _____

_____

_____

- _____

_____

_____

_____

**The "Big Points" I have to
complete today, in order to
reach my goal**

- _____

_____

- _____

_____

- _____

_____

- _____

_____

- _____

_____

- _____

_____

DAY 45

DATE

Three things I am grateful for (three new things every day)

-
-
-

What am I proud of?

What am I happy about?

Notes/Thoughts

✓ Action

Check off your "Big Points" of the morning. What did or didn't you do?

What did I learn today?

"Success is not what you have, but who you are."
—Bo Bennet

**What could I have
done better?**

_____

_____

_____

_____

_____

_____

_____

_____

**For the next 21 days,
I will...**

_____

_____

_____

_____

_____

_____

_____

In 21 days, I will...

_____

_____

_____

_____

_____

_____

✔ **Action**

Take an ice cold shower and
see how you feel afterwards.

**3 amazing things that
happened today**

- _____

_____

_____

- _____

_____

_____

- _____

_____

_____

_____

**The "Big Points" I have to
complete today, in order to
reach my goal**

- _____

_____

- _____

_____

- _____

_____

- _____

_____

- _____

_____

- _____

_____

DAY 46

DATE

Three things I am grateful for (three new things every day)

- _____
- _____
- _____

What am I proud of?

What am I happy about?

Notes/Thoughts

✅ **Action**

Check off your "Big Points" of the morning. What did or didn't you do?

What did I learn today?

"Anyone who has never made a mistake has never tried anything new."
—Albert Einstein

What could I have done better?

_____
_____
_____
_____
_____
_____
_____

For the next 20 days, I will...

_____
_____
_____
_____
_____
_____

In 20 days, I will...

_____
_____
_____
_____
_____
_____

✓ Action

"Survive" an entire day with your phone in airplane mode.

3 amazing things that happened today

- _____
  _____
  _____
- _____
  _____
  _____
- _____
  _____
  _____

The "Big Points" I have to complete today, in order to reach my goal

- _____
  _____
- _____
  _____
- _____
  _____
- _____
  _____
- _____
  _____
- _____
  _____

DAY 47

DATE

Three things I am grateful for (three new things every day)

- _____
  _____
  _____

- _____
  _____
  _____

- _____
  _____

What am I proud of?

_____
_____
_____
_____
_____
_____
_____

What am I happy about?

_____
_____
_____
_____
_____
_____

Notes/Thoughts

_____
_____
_____
_____
_____
_____

✓ Action

Check off your "Big Points" of the morning. What did or didn't you do?

"Your time is limited, don't waste it by living somebody else's life."
—Steve Jobs

What did I learn today?

_____
_____
_____
_____
_____
_____
_____
_____

What could I have done better?

_____
_____
_____
_____
_____
_____
_____

For the next 19 days, I will...

_____
_____
_____
_____
_____
_____
_____

In 19 days, I will...

_____
_____
_____
_____
_____

✔ **Action**

What is something else you loved doing as a kid? That is exactly what you will do tomorrow.

3 amazing things that happened today

- _____
  _____
  _____

- _____
  _____
  _____

- _____
  _____
  _____

The "Big Points" I have to complete today, in order to reach my goal

- _____

- _____

- _____

- _____

- _____

- _____

- _____

DAY 48

DATE

Three things I am grateful for (three new things every day)

- _____
- _____
- _____

What am I proud of?

What am I happy about?

Notes/Thoughts

✓ Action

Check off your "Big Points" of the morning. What did or didn't you do?

What did I learn today?

*"I don't stop when I am tired.
I only stop when I am done."*
—Marilyn Monroe

What could I have done better?

_____
_____
_____
_____
_____
_____
_____
_____

For the next 18 days, I will...

_____
_____
_____
_____
_____
_____

In 18 days, I will...

_____
_____
_____
_____
_____
_____

✓ Action

Borrow a skateboard and ask a skateboarder to show you how to kickflip.

3 amazing things that happened today

- _____
  _____
  _____
- _____
  _____
  _____
- _____
  _____
  _____

The "Big Points" I have to complete today, in order to reach my goal

- _____
- _____
- _____
- _____
- _____
- _____
- _____

DAY 49

DATE

Three things I am grateful for (three new things every day)

- _____
  _____
- _____
  _____
- _____
  _____

What am I proud of?

_____
_____
_____
_____
_____
_____

What am I happy about?

_____
_____
_____
_____
_____

Notes/Thoughts

_____
_____
_____
_____
_____
_____

✓ Action

Check off your "Big Points" of the morning. What did or didn't you do?

"A goal without a plan is just a wish."
—Antoine de Saint-Exupéry

What did I learn today?

_____
_____
_____
_____
_____
_____

What could I have done better?

_____
_____
_____
_____
_____
_____
_____

In 17 days, I will...

_____
_____
_____
_____
_____
_____

3 amazing things that happened today

- _____
  _____
  _____
- _____
  _____
  _____
- _____
  _____
  _____

For the next 17 days, I will...

_____
_____
_____
_____
_____
_____
_____

✓ Action

Go back to your home base
page and tell yourself your goal
and your words of joy
in front of the mirror. Enjoy!

The "Big Points" I have to complete today, in order to reach my goal

- _____
  _____
- _____
  _____
- _____
  _____
- _____
  _____
- _____
  _____
- _____

DAY 50

DATE

Three things I am grateful for (three new things every day)

- _____
  _____

- _____
  _____

- _____
  _____

What am I proud of?

_____
_____
_____
_____
_____
_____

What am I happy about?

_____
_____
_____
_____
_____
_____

Notes/Thoughts

_____
_____
_____
_____
_____
_____

Action

Check off your "Big Points" of the morning. What did or didn't you do?

"Even a step back is a step towards your goal."
—Konrad Adenauer

What did I learn today?

_____
_____
_____
_____
_____
_____

What could I have done better?

_____
_____
_____
_____
_____
_____
_____
_____

For the next 16 days, I will...

_____
_____
_____
_____
_____
_____
_____

In 16 days, I will...

_____
_____
_____
_____
_____
_____

✓ Action

Find a basketball court and hit a three-point shot.

3 amazing things that happened today

- _____
_____
_____

- _____
_____
_____

- _____
_____
_____

The "Big Points" I have to complete today, in order to reach my goal

- _____

- _____
_____

- _____
_____

- _____
_____

- _____
_____

- _____

- _____

Quarterly Meeting 3

Congratulations, you have reached 75 percent percent of your goal!

You are now heading for the last sixteen-day sprint of this unforgettable journey. You are so high up the mountain that by now you can clearly see the peak. You truly deserve deep respect!

In case your goal still seems unattainable, try changing the perspective. Although it is tempting to keep looking up toward the peak again and again, try a counterintuitive shift in your focus from results to performance. Your days are your life!

The strongest athletes all know this: Set a goal, look in the mirror. Train for six months meticulously according to your plan. Only then, you look in the mirror again. Everything else just distracts you from your goal!

Now that you've gotten this far, it's important to focus on your performance for the last sixteen days, not on your goal. Live in every "Big Point," in every step that brings you closer to your goal. Trust in the process and watch how it draws you towards your goal without you having to look up at the peak. Every new step is a compass and guides that which lives inside you and never loses its way.

Action

To help you focus on your performance, we will now integrate a talisman into your final sprint, and the final part of your journey. Find an object that speaks to you and that symbolizes a combination of strength and balance (e.g. a battery, rubber band, candle, button, etc.). On every new day, allow your talisman to remind you of the powerful combination of strength and balance. Each contraction is followed by a resting phase. Like a muscle, you will become stronger each day. Even just a single glance at your talisman is enough and will fuel your final ascent.

DAY 51

DATE

Three things I am grateful for (three new things every day)

- _____
- _____
- _____

What am I proud of?

What am I happy about?

Notes/Thoughts

✓ **Action**

Check off your "Big Points" of the morning. What did or didn't you do?

"It's not what you look at that matters, it's what you see."
—Henry David Thoreau

What did I learn today?

What could I have done better?

_____

_____

_____

_____

_____

_____

In 15 days, I will...

_____

_____

_____

_____

_____

3 amazing things that happened today

- _____

- _____

- _____

For the next 15 days, I will...

_____

_____

_____

_____

_____

_____

✅ **Action**

Before you go to bed today, go for a walk and kiss the ground with every step. If possible, walk barefoot and feel the grass, snow or sand.

The "Big Points" I have to complete today, in order to reach my goal

- _____

- _____

- _____

- _____

- _____

- _____

- _____

DAY 52

DATE

Three things I am grateful for (three new things every day)

- _____
- _____
- _____

What am I proud of?

What am I happy about?

Notes/Thoughts

> ✅ **Action**
>
> Check off your "Big Points" of the morning. What did or didn't you do?

What did I learn today?

> *"Everybody is a genius.
> But if you judge a fish by its ability to
> climb a tree, it will live its whole life
> believing that it is stupid."*
> —Albert Einstein

What could I have done better?

_____
_____
_____
_____
_____
_____
_____
_____

For the next 14 days, I will...

_____
_____
_____
_____
_____
_____

In 14 days, I will...

_____
_____
_____
_____
_____
_____

✓ **Action**

Go to the window and take ten deep breaths (in through the nose, out through the mouth).

3 amazing things that happened today

- _____
  _____
  _____
- _____
  _____
  _____
- _____
  _____
  _____

The "Big Points" I have to complete today, in order to reach my goal

- _____
  _____
- _____
  _____
- _____
  _____
- _____
  _____
- _____
  _____
- _____
  _____
- _____
  _____

DAY 53

DATE

Three things I am grateful for (three new things every day)

- _____

- _____

- _____

What am I proud of?

What am I happy about?

Notes/Thoughts

✅ **Action**

Check off your "Big Points" of the morning. What did or didn't you do?

What did I learn today?

*"I accept failure!
Everybody fails at something.
But I can't accept not trying."*
—Michael Jordan

What could I have done better?

_____
_____
_____
_____
_____
_____
_____
_____

For the next 13 days, I will...

_____
_____
_____
_____
_____
_____
_____

In 13 days, I will...

_____
_____
_____
_____
_____
_____

Action

Read in an inspiring book for ten minutes before you fall asleep.

3 amazing things that happened today

- _____
_____
_____
- _____
_____
_____
- _____
_____
_____

The "Big Points" I have to complete today, in order to reach my goal

- _____
- _____
_____
- _____
- _____
- _____
- _____
- _____

DAY 54

DATE

Three things I am grateful for (three new things every day)

- _____
- _____
- _____

What am I proud of?

What am I happy about?

Notes/Thoughts

Action

Check off your "Big Points" of the morning. What did or didn't you do?

What did I learn today?

"If you don't build your dream, someone will hire you to help build theirs."
—Tony Gaskin

What could I have done better?

_____

_____

_____

_____

_____

_____

_____

_____

For the next 12 days, I will...

_____

_____

_____

_____

_____

_____

_____

In 12 days, I will...

_____

_____

_____

_____

_____

_____

✓ Action

Call an old friend today, and ask about how they are.

3 amazing things that happened today

- _____

_____

_____

- _____

_____

_____

- _____

_____

_____

_____

The "Big Points" I have to complete today, in order to reach my goal

- _____

_____

- _____

_____

- _____

_____

- _____

_____

- _____

_____

- _____

_____

DAY 55

DATE

Three things I am grateful for (three new things every day)

-
-
-

What am I proud of?

What am I happy about?

Notes/Thoughts

✓ Action

Check off your "Big Points" of the morning. What did or didn't you do?

What did I learn today?

"Failure is the chance to start all over again, more intelligently."
—Henry Ford

What could I have done better?

_____
_____
_____
_____
_____
_____
_____
_____

For the next 11 days, I will...

_____
_____
_____
_____
_____
_____

In 11 days, I will...

_____
_____
_____
_____
_____
_____

Action

After waking up, stay in bed and smile at the ceiling for three minutes.

3 amazing things that happened today

- _____
_____
_____
- _____
_____
- _____
_____

The "Big Points" I have to complete today, in order to reach my goal

- _____
- _____
- _____
- _____
- _____
- _____
- _____

DAY 56

DATE

Three things I am grateful for (three new things every day)

- _____
- _____
- _____

What am I proud of?

What am I happy about?

Notes/Thoughts

✓ **Action**

Check off your "Big Points" of the morning. What did or didn't you do?

What did I learn today?

"The most dangerous sentence in any language is:
We've always done it this way."
—Grace Hopper

What could I have done better?

_____

_____

_____

_____

_____

_____

_____

For the next 10 days, I will...

_____

_____

_____

_____

_____

_____

In 10 days, I will...

_____

_____

_____

_____

✅ **Action**

Go without Playstation, Youtube, gaming apps or TV today.

3 amazing things that happened today

- _____

  _____

  _____

- _____

  _____

  _____

- _____

  _____

  _____

The "Big Points" I have to complete today, in order to reach my goal

- _____

- _____

- _____

- _____

- _____

- _____

- _____

DAY 57

DATE

Three things I am grateful for (three new things every day)

- _____

- _____

- _____

What am I proud of?

What am I happy about?

Notes/Thoughts

✅ **Action**

Check off your "Big Points" of the morning. What did or didn't you do?

What did I learn today?

"It is never too late to be what you might have been."
—George Eliot

What could I have done better?

_____
_____
_____
_____
_____
_____
_____

For the next 9 days, I will...

_____
_____
_____
_____
_____
_____

In 9 days, I will...

_____
_____
_____
_____
_____
_____

✅ **Action**

Go back to your home base page and tell yourself your goal and your words of joy in front of the mirror. Enjoy!

3 amazing things that happened today

- _____
  _____

- _____
  _____

- _____
  _____

The "Big Points" I have to complete today, in order to reach my goal

- _____
  _____

- _____

- _____
  _____

- _____
  _____

- _____
  _____

- _____

DAY 58

DATE

**Three things I am grateful for
(three new things every day)**

- _____
- _____
- _____

What am I proud of?

_____
_____
_____
_____
_____
_____
_____

What am I happy about?

_____
_____
_____
_____
_____
_____

Notes/Thoughts

_____
_____
_____
_____
_____
_____

✓ Action

Check off your "Big Points" of
the morning. What did or
didn't you do?

*"Doubt kills more dreams than
failure ever will."*
—Suzy Cassem

What did I learn today?

_____
_____
_____
_____
_____
_____
_____
_____

What could I have done better?

_____
_____
_____
_____
_____
_____
_____

For the next 8 days, I will...

_____
_____
_____
_____
_____
_____

In 8 days, I will...

_____
_____
_____
_____
_____
_____

✅ **Action**

Surprise a special person today with something small you cooked or baked yourself.

3 amazing things that happened today

- _____
  _____
  _____
- _____
  _____
- _____
  _____
  _____

The "Big Points" I have to complete today, in order to reach my goal

- _____
- _____
- _____
- _____
- _____
- _____
- _____

DAY 59

DATE

Three things I am grateful for (three new things every day)

- _____
  _____

- _____
  _____

- _____
  _____

What am I proud of?

_____
_____
_____
_____
_____
_____

What am I happy about?

_____
_____
_____
_____
_____

Notes/Thoughts

_____
_____
_____
_____
_____
_____

Action

Check off your "Big Points" of the morning. What did or didn't you do?

What did I learn today?

_____
_____
_____
_____
_____
_____

"To live is the rarest thing in the world. Most people exist, that is all."
—Oscar Wilde

What could I have done better?

_____

_____

_____

_____

_____

_____

_____

For the next 7 days, I will...

_____

_____

_____

_____

_____

_____

In 7 days, I will...

_____

_____

_____

_____

_____

_____

✓ **Action**

Take a different way home today and learn about new parts of your area.

3 amazing things that happened today

- _____

  _____

  _____

- _____

  _____

  _____

- _____

  _____

  _____

The "Big Points" I have to complete today, in order to reach my goal

- _____

  _____

- _____

  _____

- _____

  _____

- _____

  _____

- _____

  _____

- _____

  _____

- _____

DAY 60

/   /

DATE

Three things I am grateful for (three new things every day)

- _____
  _____

- _____
  _____

- _____
  _____

What am I proud of?

_____
_____
_____
_____
_____
_____

What am I happy about?

_____
_____
_____
_____
_____
_____

Notes/Thoughts

_____
_____
_____
_____
_____
_____

✓ Action

Check off your "Big Points" of the morning. What did or didn't you do?

What did I learn today?

_____
_____
_____
_____
_____
_____
_____

"Losers stop when they fail.
Winners fail until they succeed."
—Robert Kiyosaki

What could I have done better?

_____
_____
_____
_____
_____
_____
_____
_____

For the next 6 days, I will...

_____
_____
_____
_____
_____
_____
_____

In 6 days, I will...

_____
_____
_____
_____
_____
_____

✓ **Action**

Buy movie tickets and
go to see a comedy with
someone special today.

3 amazing things that happened today

• _____
  _____
  _____
• _____
  _____
  _____
• _____
  _____
  _____
  _____

The "Big Points" I have to complete today, in order to reach my goal

• _____
  _____
• _____
  _____
• _____
  _____
• _____
  _____
• _____
  _____
• _____
  _____

DAY 61

DATE

Three things I am grateful for (three new things every day)

- _____
  _____
  _____

- _____
  _____
  _____

- _____
  _____

What am I proud of?

_____
_____
_____
_____
_____
_____
_____

What am I happy about?

_____
_____
_____
_____
_____
_____
_____

Notes/Thoughts

_____
_____
_____
_____
_____
_____

✓ **Action**

Check off your "Big Points" of the morning. What did or didn't you do?

What did I learn today?

_____
_____
_____
_____
_____
_____
_____

"The only place success comes before work is in the dictionary."
—Vidal Sassoon

What could I have done better?

_____

_____

_____

_____

_____

_____

_____

_____

In 5 days, I will...

_____

_____

_____

_____

_____

_____

3 amazing things that happened today

- _____

_____

_____

- _____

_____

_____

- _____

_____

_____

For the next 5 days, I will...

_____

_____

_____

_____

_____

_____

✔ **Action**

Smile at a stranger today.

The "Big Points" I have to complete today, in order to reach my goal

- _____

- _____

- _____

- _____

- _____

- _____

- _____

DAY 62

DATE

Three things I am grateful for (three new things every day)

- _____
- _____
- _____

What am I proud of?

What am I happy about?

Notes/Thoughts

✅ **Action**

Check off your "Big Points" of the morning. What did or didn't you do?

What did I learn today?

"Success is not final,
failure is not fatal:
it is the courage to continue that counts."
— Winston Churchill

What could I have done better?

_____

_____

_____

_____

_____

_____

_____

For the next 4 days, I will...

_____

_____

_____

_____

_____

_____

In 4 days, I will...

_____

_____

_____

_____

_____

✓ Action

Drink three liters of
flat water today.

3 amazing things that happened today

- _____

  _____

  _____

- _____

  _____

  _____

- _____

  _____

  _____

The "Big Points" I have to complete today, in order to reach my goal

- _____

- _____

- _____

- _____

- _____

- _____

- _____

DAY 63

DATE

Three things I am grateful for (three new things every day)

- _____
  _____
- _____
  _____
- _____
  _____

What am I proud of?

_____
_____
_____
_____
_____
_____
_____

What am I happy about?

_____
_____
_____
_____
_____
_____
_____

Notes/Thoughts

_____
_____
_____
_____
_____
_____

✓ Action

Check off your "Big Points" of the morning. What did or didn't you do?

What did I learn today?

_____
_____
_____
_____
_____
_____
_____

"f you do not like something, change it;
If you can't change it,
change the way you think about it."
— Mary Engelbreit

What could I have done better?

_____
_____
_____
_____
_____
_____
_____
_____

For the next 3 days, I will...

_____
_____
_____
_____
_____
_____
_____

In 3 days, I will...

_____
_____
_____
_____
_____
_____

✅ **Action**

Apologize to
someone today.

3 amazing things that happened today

- _____
  _____
  _____
- _____
  _____
  _____
- _____
  _____
  _____
  _____

The "Big Points" I have to complete today, in order to reach my goal

- _____
- _____
- _____
- _____
- _____
- _____

DAY 64

DATE

Three things I am grateful for (three new things every day)

- _____
- _____
- _____

What am I proud of?

What am I happy about?

Notes/Thoughts

✅ **Action**

Check off your "Big Points" of the morning. What did or didn't you do?

*"Peace comes from within.
Do not seek it without."*
— Buddha

What did I learn today?

**What could I have
done better?**

_____
_____
_____
_____
_____
_____
_____
_____

In 2 days, I will...

_____
_____
_____
_____
_____
_____

**For the next 2 days,
I will...**

_____
_____
_____
_____
_____
_____

✅ **Action**

Ask an older person about
an important life lesson today.

**3 amazing things that
happened today**

- _____
_____
_____
- _____
_____
_____
- _____
_____
_____

**The "Big Points" I have to
complete today, in order to
reach my goal**

- _____
- _____
- _____
- _____
- _____
- _____
- _____

DAY 65

DATE

Three things I am grateful for (three new things every day)

- _____
- _____
- _____

What am I proud of?

What am I happy about?

Notes/Thoughts

✅ Action

Check off your "Big Points" of the morning. What did or didn't you do?

What did I learn today?

"You must be the change you wish to see in the world."
— Mahatma Gandhi

What could I have done better?

_____
_____
_____
_____
_____
_____
_____

For the next 1 days, I will...

_____
_____
_____
_____
_____
_____

In 1 days, I will...

_____
_____
_____
_____
_____

✔ **Action**

Go back to your home base page and tell yourself your goal and your words of joy in front of the mirror. Enjoy!

3 amazing things that happened today

- _____
_____
_____
- _____
_____
_____
- _____
_____
_____
_____

The "Big Points" I have to complete today, in order to reach my goal

- _____
- _____
- _____
- _____
- _____
- _____
- _____

DAY 66

DATE

Three things I am grateful for (three new things every day)

- _____

- _____

- _____

What am I proud of?

What am I happy about?

Notes/Thoughts

✅ **Action**

Check off your "Big Points" of the morning. What did or didn't you do?

What did I learn today?

"If you light a lamp for somebody, it will also brighten your path."
— Buddha

What could I have done better?

_____

_____

_____

_____

_____

_____

_____

Today, I will...

_____

_____

_____

_____

_____

_____

_____

Today, I have...

_____

_____

_____

_____

_____

_____

✓ **Action**

"Survive" an entire day with your phone in airplane mode.

3 amazing things that happened today

- _____

  _____

  _____

- _____

  _____

  _____

- _____

  _____

  _____

  _____

The "Big Points" I have to complete today, in order to reach my goal

- _____

  _____

- _____

  _____

- _____

  _____

- _____

  _____

- _____

  _____

- _____

  _____

Quarterly Meeting 4—Celebration

You have reached your goal!

People rarely finish what they start. As of today, you have proven to yourself that you have what only a few people have, as you are willing to do what only few people do.

Today, you have finally reached the top of the mountain! So, enjoy the breathtaking view, look back into the valley, and reflect down the path you have traveled using time, discipline, strength, and passion.

Inhale trust and exhale fear.

Now, from this new vantage point, high atop your peak performance, lift your eyes one more time to realize that there are still so many more peaks to climb. You're not there yet, you never are. When the eyes are ready, the rest of the path appears. Life is not about discovery, it's about creation. Keep going and the path becomes the goal.

Every step of this journey, every page in this journal, was not only about reaching a goal, it was the unique opportunity to introduce you to the person you have become during the journey.

This was just the beginning. What mountains are you going to climb next?

Take a minute, smile inside, be proud and truly thankful for this moment—this moment is the reason this journal found you!

• Notes •

• About the Author •

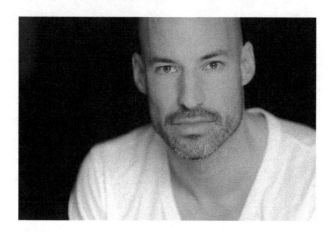

Matthew Mockridge studied international business and management at Florida International University in Miami, Florida, USA. He is a serial entrepreneur, a bestselling author, an official coach to the contestants in the primetime TV show START-UP!, and an international keynote speaker for companies such as Philips, Sony Pictures Television, Lufthansa, RE/MAX, and many more.

www.matthewmockridge.com

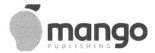

Mango Publishing, established in 2014, publishes an eclectic list of books by diverse authors—both new and established voices—on topics ranging from business, personal growth, women's empowerment, LGBTQ studies, health, and spirituality to history, popular culture, time management, decluttering, lifestyle, mental wellness, aging, and sustainable living. We were recently named 2019's #1 fastest growing independent publisher by Publishers Weekly. Our success is driven by our main goal, which is to publish high quality books that will entertain readers as well as make a positive difference in their lives.

Our readers are our most important resource; we value your input, suggestions, and ideas. We'd love to hear from you—after all, we are publishing books for you!

Please stay in touch with us and follow us at:
Facebook: Mango Publishing
Twitter: @MangoPublishing
Instagram: @MangoPublishing
LinkedIn: Mango Publishing
Pinterest: Mango Publishing

Sign up for our newsletter at www.mangopublishinggroup.com and receive a free book!